Low Carb:

21 Delicious And Mouth Watering Recipes For Guaranteed Weight Loss

-RAGHAV GIRDHAR AND NEERAJ SOLANKI

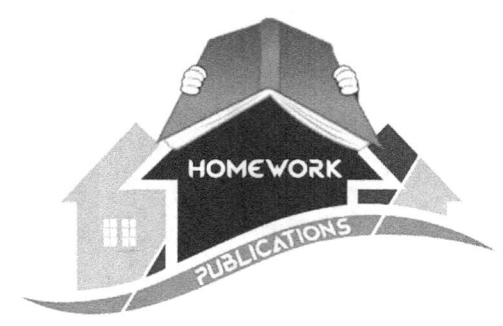

THANK YOU FOR BUYING HOMEWORK PUBLICATION EBOOK

BE IN CONTACT WITH US TO UPDATE YOURSELF WITH OUR UPCOMING BOOK "BULLETPROOF DIET".

EMAIL:

NEERAJ SOLANKI: mailto:neerajkumarsolanki@gmail.com

RAGHAV GIRDHAR: mailto:raghavgirdhar7007@gmail.com

DISCLAIMER:

INDEX

3. <u>Thaiodin chicken & mixture mush-room</u>

4. <u>Pizzianno Frittata</u>

5. <u>Master chef's Chicken Papri-kash</u>

6. <u>Sweet Green potato & Sage Soup</u>

7. <u>Turkey Mozzarella-bursted Hamburgers</u>

INTRODUCTION

Diets are the most popular and attention gaining subject in this planet, People are concerned about the food they are eating. it is truth that you become what you eat! Now that time when people loved unhealthy tasty food is over now everyone wants to take care of his or her beautiful physique. this new trend involves the combination of healthy ingredients and healthy food. time was gone when proteins and vegetables were the enemy.

Tired of getting results of normal common dieting food? It's time for a big change and you have stepped to exact place. this book focuses on one of the most experienced low carb diet invented ever or we can say the realistic diet. No more useless tips of weight loss, no more calorie counting every day, no more starvation! with this low carb diet none of these thing are needed! instead the low carb diet is applying limits on the amount of carbohydrates ingested and investing more in food that are high in proteins and fat. this diet comes with the surety of weight loss. but it can help you mind and body in general terms of health as well.

Carbohydrates, also known as carbs, are the type of calorie-container and provider macronutrient which are being found in many foods and beverages. The main species of carbs are generally found in grains which are hard and slow to digest, But Carbs are also in fruits, vegetables, nuts and milk. However these types of carbohydrates digest easier and faster than those which are found in grains and are used over those which are found in grains.

Carbs are the essential source of fuel and energy for your body and mind. The carbs get broke down into sugars and starches and then absorbed into blood stream where they reach the cell after spiking the sugar level. when sugar level of your body increases, you body releases insulin which allows the cells to absorb sugars. This leads to weight gain and that is opposite of what fat burn fat for energy rather than using sugar as fuel. A low carbs diet focuses on proteins fish eggs fruits no starchy vegetables and the dairy products. This excludes: breads, grains, pasta, seeds and nuts certain deserts.

This book is a proof that a low carbs is a joy and includes only the mouth watering delicious foods made using very easy to understand and follow recipes.

BREAKFAST

1. EGGIE VEGIE

What can be better than having lots of protein, vitamins and minerals without having carbs or fat. This dish is perfect to start the day. It keeps your tummy full for long time

Ingredients:

- Coconut oil,
- Spinach,
- Frozen Vegetable Mix (carrots, cauliflower, broccoli, green beans,)
- Spices
- Eggs

Instructions:

1. 1.First put some coconut oil in the frying pan and heat it for some time.
2. Add vegetables like green beans, carrots, cauliflowers, broccoli, and whatever you want. Let it cook at some heat for some time.
3. Add eggs as per your requirement.(I took 3).
4. 4 now add spices mix, although salt and pepper gives great taste.
5. Add some spinach.
6. Stir the mix in frying pan and heat it until ready.

2. Grilled Chicken Wings With Veggies

This is one of my favorite breakfast meal. Vegetables around grilled chicken wings, awesome and yummy.

Ingredients:

- Chicken Wings,
- Spices,
- Green vegetables,
- Salsa.

Instructions:

1. Put some of the spices like salt and pepper on chicken wings.
2. Put it in oven for some time, and heat it at 180-200 degree Fahrenheit for about 40 minutes.
3. Grill it until the chicken wings become brown in color and crunchy.
4. At last serve it worth some vegetables and salsa.

3. Eggs And Bacon

According to me bacon is a healthy food as it is a processed meat. It contains low carbs so this can be added to your low carbs diet and can help to lose weight. I would say to eat it twice or thrice in a week.

Ingredients:

- Bacon,
- Eggs
- Sea salt, garlic powder and onion powder (according to taste)

Instructions:

1. Put some oil in frying pan and heat it.
2. Add bacon to pan and fry until it ready.
3. Now put the bacon on the plate and fry 4 eggs in the bacon fat.
4. You can add up some flavor to the eggs by adding some sea salt, garlic powder and onion powder to them at the time of frying.

4. Ground Beef With Spinach and spices

Ground beef with spinach and spices is one of the best meal to have in breakfast. And it's perfect if someone have spare ground beef laying around.

Ingredients:

- Coconut Oil,
- Onions,
- Ground Beef,
- Spinach,
- Salt, Pepper
- Bell Pepper.

Instructions:

1. Cut 2-3 onion in very small pieces first.
2. Now put coconut oil in frying pan, and turn up the heat.
3. Add onion to the frying pan, and stir it time to time for minute or two.
4. Now add ground beef to it.
5. Add spices like salt and pepper according to taste.
6. Add spinach to it.
7. Stir for some time, fry until ready, serve with a sliced bell pepper.

5. <u>Cheeseburgers Without The Bun</u>

You will never get tired of this meal. It's sound great 'Burgers without bun' isn't it. It is made with some cheese and can be served with spinach.

Ingredients:

- Butter,
- Hamburgers,
- Cheddar Cheese,
- Cream Cheese,
- Salsa,
- Spices,
- Spinach.

Instructions:
1. First of all put some butter on pan, and turn up the heat.
2. After that add burger and spices into it.
3. Now it's time to flip until close to being ready.
4. Add few slices of cheddar and cream cheese on top of it.
5. Lower the heat and put the lid until the cheese melts.
6. U can serve it with raw spinach.
7. Add some salsa on the top to make the burgers more juicy.

6. Chicken breast

Eating chicken breast alone is tasteless so I do lots of butter to make them palatable.

Ingredients:

- Butter,
- Chicken Breast,
- Salt,
- Pepper,
- Garlic Powder,
- Curry

Instructions:

1. First step is to cut the chicken breast.
2. Now add some butter to pan and turn up the heat.
3. It's time to add chicken pieces.
4. Once you are done with adding chicken pieces, add some salt, pepper and garlic powder to it.
5. Stir it well until the chicken pieces turns brown and gets texture.
6. Serve it with some green vegetable.
   1.

7. Meatsu Fake Meat-Based Pizza...

All pizza lovers, surely you going to love this. Try at home. It's a new modified form of non-veg pizza. In this you can add up ingredients like vegetables, mushrooms, cheese and anything what you want.

Ingredients:

- Ground Beef,
- Salsa,
- Onions,
- Spice,
- Garlic Powder,
- Shredded Cheese and
- Bacon.

Instructions:

1. At first u have to cut onions and bacon into small pieces.
2. Then you have to mix onions, salsa, ground beef, garlic powder, and spices.
3. Add cheese(shredded) on the top.
4. Now it's time to spread bacon pieces over it.
5. After doing all this, put it into oven and heat it at180-200°C (356-392°F) for about 30-40 min, till the cheese and bacon looks crunchy.

LUNCH

1. <u>Grilled Marinated Shrimp</u>

"The super easy way of making a delicious shrimp of marinade so that you don't even have to apply cocktail sauce! Cayenne pepper scare you always right? Don't let it to do so. Children love to have shrimp more than their parents! It is also not very difficult to make. Just make it with the use of fresh or frozen shrimp and use an indoor electric grill if the weather is not good for outside grilling. Serve it with baked potato, salad and garlic bread. you will not get disappointed!!!"

Ingredients

- 1/3 cup olive oil
- 1/4 teaspoon cayenne pepper
- 1/4 cup tomato sauce
- 2 tablespoons red wine vinegar
- 1/2 teaspoon salt
- 2 tablespoons chopped fresh basil
- 3 cloves garlic, minced
- 2 pounds fresh shrimp, peeled and deveined
- skewers

Total time: 60 mins

Procedure

1. Take a bowl and add some garlic and stir it together with oil of olive, red wine vinegar and tomato sauce now season it with cayenne pepper and salt. Take another small bowl and add shrimp

to the second bowl and stir until it gets coated evenly . cover and refrigerate for 35 to 60 minutes, stir it twice.

2. Preheat the grill for heat. Take skewers threaded by shrimp, pierce it once near the tail and do it once near the head. Remove the marinade.

3. Grill grate lightly oil. Cook shrimp on grill which is preheated for 3 to 4 minutes both sides, or until it gets opaque.

2. Little Spinach White Omelet

"Tender Parmesan cheese, little spinach and a baby nutmeg are cooked with eggs. This can also be called as a carbs-cutter's perfect start for a perfect day."

Ingredients

- 2 eggs
- 1/8 teaspoon ground nutmeg
- 1/4 teaspoon onion powder
- 1 1/2 tablespoons grated Parmesan cheese
- 1 cup torn baby spinach leaves

Total Time: 18 mins

Procedure

1. Take a small bowl and beat eggs into it, stir it properly
2. Then add spinach and parmesan cheese. Do some seasoning with nut mug onion powder, pepper and salt.
3. Take a small medium heated and cooking sprayed coated skillet, put the mixture of eggs and cook it completely for 3 mins to make it partially set.
4. Flip it with spatula and keep cooking for 3-4 mins. Decrease heat to low and keep it cooking for 3-4 mins, or to desired requirement.

3. Chicken Pot Top Crocked

This recipe is by far the most delicious recipe comes under the niche of chicken. it takes some time but yes it comes in the lowest most carb containing recipes.

Ingredients:

- 1/2 teaspoon black pepper
- 1 teaspoon cayenne pepper
- 1 teaspoon thyme
- 4 teaspoons salt
- 1 teaspoon white pepper
- 1 teaspoon onion powder
- 2 teaspoons paprika
- 1 large roasting chicken (with pop-up timer if possible)
- 1/2 teaspoon garlic powder
-
- 1 cup chopped onion

Total Time: 20 hrs

Procedure

1. Take a small bowl, combine or mix the spices properly.
2. Remove any giblets from chicken and make sure that chicken is purely clean.
3. Rub spice mixture onto the chicken.

4. Place in releasable plastic bag and refrigerate it whole night.
5. When it gets ready to cook, put chopped onion in the bottom of the crock pot.
6. Add chicken to it. Now no liquid is needed, the chicken will make its own juices by its own.
7. Cook on low 5-8 hours.

4. <u>Asparagus And Chicken Fry</u>

Asparagus is one of my favorite spring vegetables, and this recipe is very quick stir-fry with chicken, garlic, ginger and lemon, can make your weeknight meal great. You can also serve this over rice to make your meal complete.

Ingredients:

- 1 1/2 pounds chicken breast
- Kosher salt
- 1/2 cup reduced-sodium chicken broth
- 2 tablespoons reduced-sodium soya 2 tablespoons water
- 1 tbsp canola or grape seed oil
- 1 bunch asparagus, cut into 2-inch pieces
- 6 cloves garlic, chopped
- 1 tbsp fresh ginger
- 3 tablespoons fresh lemon juice
- fresh black pepper, to taste

Procedure

1. Season the chicken with salt and combine chicken broth with soy sauce in a bowl.
2. Take a medium nonstick wok and put it at medium high heat. When it heats properly add 1 teaspoon of the oil, now add asparagus and cook about 3-4 minutes. Add spices like garlic ginger and cook about 1 min until it turns golden.

3. It's time to increase the heat to high, and add 1 teaspoon of oil with half of the chicken and cook for 4 minutes on each side until it become brown. Do the same with another half of the chicken.

4. Now the soy sauce mixture is added and is cooked for 1-1/2 minutes. It's time to add cornstarch mixture and lemon juice and stir well. When it simmers. Remove the chicken and asparagus from the heat and serve.

5. Salad Of Chickpea And Salmon

We have to try seafood instead of meat as salmon and other seafoods are very rich in good nutrients. Adding salmon with chickpeas, dill and vegetables and fruits can make this dish very nutritive and cool. This can be enjoyed in everyday's lunch, and you will never get bored of it.

Ingredients

- 2 cloves of garlic, finely minced
- 5 stalks of celery, thinly sliced
- 3 shallots, finely minced
- 2 bell peppers, thinly sliced
- 1 pint tomatoes, halved
- ½ cup of olive oil
- 1 large cucumber, halved and sliced
- 1 tablespoon red wine vinegar
- 1 teaspoon kosher salt
- 2 cans chickpeas, rinsed and drained
- juice and zest from 1 lemon
- ½ teaspoon freshly ground black pepper
- ½ teaspoon smoked paprika
- 1 teaspoon fresh or dried dill
- ½ teaspoon ground cumin
- ½ teaspoon crushed red pepper flakes
- 2-3 cans salmon, drained

Total Time: 1 hour 15 mins

Procedure

1. Chop and mince the celery, garlic, bell peppers, cucumber and tomatoes. Now, olive oil, lemon juice and zest, black pepper, paprika, salt, dill, red wine vinegar, cumin and crushed red pepper flakes are tossed together.
2. Add salmon to the bowl. Toss it to combine with mixture. Saturate the salad and put it in the refrigerator. Adjust seasoning if required.
3. Serve it.
4. It can be eaten for 4 days if it is put in an air tight container and is placed in refrigerator.

6. Shiitake Mushrooms With Goat Cheese Steak Salad

what will happen if you will have to eat beef for the whole week, obviously you will get bored. but if you can adjust with a little change you are going to enjoy this. the meaty flavor and texture of shitake mushrooms is when paired with tangy goat cheese went well with beef.

Ingredients

- 150g leftover cooked roast beef
- 2 cups mixed greens
- 100g fresh shiitake mushrooms
- 30g no ripened soft goat cheese
- 1-2 tbsp balsamic vinegar
- Lime juice to taste
- Pinch freshly cracked black pepper

Instructions

1. Cook the sliced shitake mushrooms in a non stick pan at medium high heat for 3-4 minutes per side.
2. Now you have to slice roast beef as thin as you can.
3. Now you have to place the mixed greens at the bottom of the shallow plate.
4. Put slice of beef in the center of the pile of greens in a manner so that it looks good.
5. Now you have to add soft goat cheese and shitake mushrooms.
6. Drizzle some lemon juice and vinegar for taste.
7. Sprinkle black pepper.

7. Salad Of Chicken, Palm And Avocado

I will highly recommend this salad to lazy people or busy people. Its easy to make, tasty, fresh and healthful plus nutritive too.

Ingredients

- For the Salad
  1 bone-in, skin-on chicken breast
  Olive oil
  Salt and pepper
  One 14-ounce can hearts of palm, cut into chunks (about 1 1/3 cups)
  1 cup frozen corn kernels, thawed under running water and drained
  3 roasted red peppers, washed well and drained, then cut into bite-sized pieces
  2 ripe avocados, cut in half, pit removed, cut in a cross hatch then scooped out
  Cilantro for garnish

- For the Vinaigrette
  2 teaspoons apple cider vinegar
  1 tablespoon fresh squeezed lime juice (about half a lime)
  1/2 teaspoon Dijon mustard
  2 tablespoons olive oil
  2 tablespoons vegetable oil
  ¾ teaspoon kosher or sea salt, or more to taste
  ¼ teaspoon oregano
  1 scallion, white and light green parts, sliced
  1/2 teaspoon honey
  ¼ teaspoon freshly ground black pepper

1. Heat the oven at around 400°F. Place the washed and dried chicken on a parchment. Sprinkle some salt and pepper and drizzle with olive oil. Now bake it for 30-35 minutes. Cool it completely for at least 1 hour. You can eat it for some days by putting into the refrigerator.

2. Clean the chicken after removing bone. Now cut it into pieces and put it into large bowl. Add red pepper, avocado, corn and hearts of

3. Take another bowl to make the vinaigrette: whisk lemon juice, mustard and vinegar together. Now drizzle in both oils slowly, whisk it. Now salt, scallion,, pepper, honey and oregano is combined.

4. Pour vinaigrette over the salad and toss gently. Serve with cilantro.

DINNER

1. Bursting Mushroom cake

Ingredients:

- 1 cup Italian-style dried bread crumbs
- 1 cup grated Pecorino Romano
- 4 garlic cloves, peeled and minced
- 4 tablespoons fresh Italian parsley leaves (chopped)
- 1/6 cup extra-virgin olive oil
- 2 tablespoon mint (chopped) leaves and Salt
- freshly ground black pepper
- 38 large (2 1/2-inch-diameter) white mushrooms

Total Time: 38 min

Procedure:

1. Firstly Preheat the microwave oven to 410 degrees F.

2. Put the bread crumbs, Stir the crumbs, Pecorino Romano, garlic, salt and pepper, parsley, mint, to taste, and 4 tbsp olive oil in a large bowl to blend completely.

3. Fill a heavy large baking sheet with near around 2 tbsp olive oil to cover.

4. Mix the filling into the mushroom cavities and set it on the baking sheet, remember t arrange in an order to get cavity side up. Sprinkle the remaining oil over the made filling in each of the mushroom.

5. Bake it until the mushrooms get tendered and the filling is heated through and golden on top, near around 25-26 minutes. Serve and enjoy.

2. Vitamin C-Dried Goat and Tomato Cheese Skewers

Ingredients:

- 1 (8-ounce) (chilled) log goat cheese
- 1/2 bunch fresh basil leaves
- 20 sun-dried tomatoes packed in oil
- 1 cup pistachio nuts, finely chopped
- 20 sun-dried tomatoes packed in oil
- Extra requirement: Special equipment: 20 small skewers or cocktail toothpicks

Total Time: 18-20 min

Procedure:

- Fill a jar with steamed water. Dip a knife into the hot water and cut the goat cheese log into slices in half lengthwise. remember to Slice each half of the goat slice into 10 pieces making sure that to dip the knife into the hot water in between slicing to ensure a nice clean cut. Roll each piece of goat cheese to convert it into balls approximately 1/2-inch in diameter and put onto a sheet of cookie which is lined with waxed paper.
- Add chopped pistachio nuts to a medium bowl. Roll a goat cheese ball to turn it into the pistachio nuts and coat 1/2 of the ball. Get back to the sheet pan and repeat with the remaining goat cheese balls.
- Drain out the oil from the tomatoes and put it onto a plate lined with a paper towel.

- Skewer a goat cheese ball onto the skewer. Lay a basil leaf on the top of a sun-dried tomato. Fold the tomato around the basil leaf in half and add to the skewer with the cheese of goat. Repeat it with remaining skewers. Arrange on a serving container, cover and keep in the refrigerator until it gets ready to serve.

3. Thaiodin chicken & mixture mush-room

Ingredients

- 1 tbsp Thai red curry paste
- zest and juice 2 limes
- 2 tsp sugar
- 1 tbsp Thai fish sauce
- 1l hot chicken stock
- 100g Portobello mushrooms, sliced
- bunch spring onions, sliced, whites and greens seperated
- 200g leftover chicken, shredded

Total time- 15-18 mins

Procedure

- Dip the tip of the stock into a saucepan, then make a curry paste and stir into it, sugar, lime juice, fish sauce and most of the zest. Let it come to the boiling stage, then add the whites of the spring onion and mushrooms into it. Cover, then do it on same for 2 minutes.
- Stir properly in the most of the spring onion greens chicken and heat it gently, then take some bowls and serve ladled scattered with remaining zest lime. serve with lime juice (extra) fish sauce and sugar on the side so that everyone can get the taste of their own demand.

4. <u>Pizzianno Frittata</u>

Ingredients

- 12 eggs
- 1/2 cup grated parmigiano-reggiano
- 1 teaspoon hot sauce, such as Tabasco
- Salt and pepper
- 2 cloves garlic, chopped
- 3 tablespoons grated onion
- 1 cup whole milk or half-and-half
- 1/4 cup dry red wine
- A small handful (chopped) flat-leaf parsley
- 1/4 cup EVOO
- 1 cup crushed tomatoes
- 1/4 pound hot pepperoni, must be finely chopped, or (for vegetarian option) 2 Fresno chili peppers sliced
- 1 sprig oregano, or 1/2 tsp. oregano (dried &finely chopped)
- 6 ounces fresh mozzarella, shredded on the large side of a box grated or thinly sliced
- A few leaves fresh basil, torn

Procedure

- Firstly preheat the microwave oven to 410 degrees F. take a large bowl and beat the eggs into it mix it with milk , salt and pepper, hot sauce, parimigiano-reggiano.

- In a comparatively large ovenproof pan, heat 2 tablespoons EVOO over medium to medium- high heat. mix the eggs and keep stirring and settling them as they cook. when the eggs starts to firm up, transfer the skillet to the oven. Bake until it gets light golden and gets puffed but not cooked through, near about 10-12 minutes.
- Meanwhile, in another skillet, heat the left 2 tablespoons EVOO over medium heat. Add the chilies, onion, garlic and oregano and cook, stir it properly, for 3 to 4 minutes. Add the wine and cook to reduce it slightly, you can do it for 1 minute, its enough. Add the tomatoes and low it to the chicken, for 10-12 mins.
- Remove the frittata from the oven and top with the mozzarella and tomato sauce. to melt the cheese bake it for 10-12 minutes. Top with the parsley and basil.

5. Master chef's Chicken Papri-kash

Amazing red paprika, this recipe is the main seasoning in the cooking manner of Hungarians, and it gives this light version of chicken paprikash its color. Do change the heat by using hot, sweet or a mixture of paprikash. Serve over wet egg noodles with a side of cool fruit salad for dessert and steamed broccoli.

Ingredients

- 1 pound boneless, skinless chicken breasts, cut into 2-inch pieces (trimmed)
- 1/4 teaspoon kosher salt
- 2 large green bell peppers, thinly sliced
- 1/2 cup dry white wine
- 2 tablespoons chopped fresh parsley
- 2 teaspoons hot or sweet paprika
- 1 large onion, halved and thinly sliced
- 1/4 teaspoon freshly ground pepper
- 1 tablespoon canola oil
- 1/4 cup reduced-fat sour cream
- 1 1/2 cups canned crushed tomatoes
- 1 tablespoon lemon juice
- 1/2 cup reduced-sodium chicken broth

Time: 45 minutes

Procedure

- Take a vessel and put chicken into Vessel, sprinkle pepper and salt on the chicken. Heat the oil in a big pan over medium-high heat. add chicken to it and cook it properly. turn it occasionally, until it gets browned, 4to 5 minutes. transfer the chicken to a bowl o a plate
- Add bell peppers and onion to the skillet and cook it properly, should be covered, over a medium heat, stir it occasionally, let it be soft and smooth, near about 4-5 minutes. add paprika and cook it well, until it gives you a descent fragrance. around 30-35 seconds. add wine to it, increase heat to between medium high and cook it well , stir it properly, until 80 percent of it gets evaporated, about 1-1/2 minutes, add broth, tomatoes and lemon juice. boil it. Return the chicken and any accumulated juices to the pan, reduce heat to low. add some sauce over the chicken and cook it well and turn it occasionally, until the chicken is cooked through, near around 7 to 10 mins.
- Remove it from the heat, stir in the sour cream. Sprinkle it with parsley.

6. <u>Sweet Green potato & Sage Soup</u>

This kale-and-spinach soup has a amazing complex nature. It's slightly sweet, with a bright note of lemon and the subtle aromatics of thyme, garlic and sage. Japanese yams are beautifully flavorful; they have a snow-white inside and dark purplish skin. Ask for them to your farmers' market or grocery, but you don't get it, substitute it with regular sweet potatoes.

Ingredients

- 3 tablespoons (divided) extra-virgin olive oil plus more for garnish
- 2 large onions, chopped
- 2 tablespoons plus (divided) 4 cups water
- 1 teaspoon salt, divided
- 1 teaspoon fresh thyme leaves (chopped) or 1/2 (dried) teaspoon
- 1 large bunch Tuscan, lacinato or Russian kale
- 14 cups gently packed spinach ,any tough stems (trimmed)
- 4 cloves garlic, sliced
- 2 medium or 1 large Japanese yam or sweet potato (about 1 1/4 pounds)
- 4 cups vegetable broth, store-bought or homemade
- 8 sage leaves or 1 teaspoon crumbled dried
- 1 tablespoon agave nectar, or more to taste (optional)
- Pinch of cayenne pepper
- 1 tablespoon fresh lemon juice, or more to taste
- Freshly ground pepper to taste
- 16 fried sage leaves for garnish

Time: 1 hour

Procedure

- Heat 2 tablespoons oil in a large pan over medium to high heat. Add onions and 1/4 teaspoon salt; cook it well, stir it frequently, until the onions are starting to get brown, about 4 to 5 minutes. Reduce the heat to low, stir in 2 tablespoons water, garlic, thyme and cover. Cook it well, stir it frequently until the pan cools down, and then do it occasionally, always cover the pan again, until the onions are totally reduced and have a deep caramel color, it takes for about 30 to 35 minutes.
- Meanwhile, remove ribs and tough stems from kale and coarsely chop the greens. Peel sweet potato and dice into 1-inch pieces. Coarsely chop spinach; set it aside.
- Mix the remaining 3/4 teaspoon salt and 4 cups water in a soup pot or Dutch the oven; add the kale, sweet potato and sage. Bring it to a boil. Reduce the heat to maintain a simmer, then cover and cook it for 15-18 minutes.
- Stir in the spinach, return back to a simmer, cover and cook it well, stir it once halfway through, for 10-12 minutes more. When the onions are filled with caramel, stir simmering liquid into them
- Mix them with the soup. Add broth, return to a simmer, cover and cook it well for 5-6 minutes more.
- Puree the soup in the pot with an immersion blender until perfectly smooth or in a regular blender in batches (return it to the pot). Stir in cayenne, a 1 tbsp lemon juice and few grinds of pepper. If the soup is sweet to your taste, add more lemon juice; if it tarts too much, add agave nectar, if desired. Just before serving, whisk the 1 remaining tablespoon oil into the soup. Garnish every bowl of soup with a sprinkle of oil and 2 fried sage leaves.

7. Turkey Mozzarella-bursted Hamburgers

These tasty turkey burgers, dressed with marinara sauce and served on toasted focaccia, are reminiscent of a pizza sausage . Shredded mozzarella when combined with fresh basil melts beautifully inside these gems.

Ingredients

Marinara sauce

- 2 teaspoons extra-virgin olive oil
- 4 cloves garlic, minced
- 1 small onion, finely chopped
- 2 cups chopped plum tomatoes, with juices
- 1/2 teaspoon salt
- 6 sun-dried tomatoes(oil-packed), drained and chopped finely
- 2 tablespoons chopped fresh basil
- 1/2 teaspoon freshly ground pepper

Burgers

- 1 pound 93%-lean ground turkey
- 1/4 cup finely chopped scallions
- 2 teaspoons minced garlic
- 2 tablespoons fresh basil (finely chopped)

- 2 teaspoons extra-virgin olive oil1 teaspoon freshly grated lemon zest

- 1/2 teaspoon dried oregano2 teaspoons Worcestershire sauce1/4 teaspoon salt
- 1/2 cup shredded part-skim divided mozzarella cheese
- 4 4-inch-square slices foccacia bread, (about 2 ounces each), toasted
- 1/2 teaspoon freshly ground pepper

Preparation

- Firstly to prepare marinara sauce: Heat 2 tablespoons oil in a medium saucepan over medium heat. Add garlic and onion, cover and cook well, stir it frequently, until it gets translucent, 5 to 8 minutes. Stir it in fresh tomatoes and any juices, sun-dried tomatoes, 1/2 teaspoon pepper and 1/2 teaspoon salt. Bring to a simmer and cook it well, stir it occasionally, until the tomatoes get broken down, it will take 10 minutes. Stir in basil and remove it from the heat. Then transfer to a food processor and pulse to form a coarse-textured sauce. Return to the pan and set it aside.
- To prepare burgers: Place turkey, garlic, scallions, Worcestershire sauce, oregano, lemon zest, 1/2 teaspoon pepper and 1/4 teaspoon salt in a large bowl and gently combine it, without over mixing it, until evenly incorporated. Form into 8 thin patties about 4 inches wide and 3/8 inch thick.
- Combine basil and 1/4 cup cheese and place an equal amount in the center of 4 patties. Cover it with the remaining patties and crimp its edges closed.
- Heat 2 teaspoons oil in a large nonstick skillet over medium heat. Add burgers and cook it well, turning once, until an instant-read

thermometer inserted in the center registers 165°F, 8 to 10 minutes total.

- Warm the marinara on the stove. While assembling the burgers, spread 3 tablespoons of marinara on each toasted focaccia, top it with a burger, about 3 more tablespoons of marinara and 1 tablespoon of the remaining cheese.
- Grilling Variation: To grill the turkey burgers, firstly preheat a grill to medium. Do oiling of the grill rack. Grill the patties, turn it once, until an read thermometer inserted in the center registers 165°F, 10 minutes total.

<u>ENJOY</u>

If you enjoyed the recipes of this book, please share your thoughts about book . And ask your friends and relatives to read it once. If you would encourage us this will help us to make us to serve you better. We would be very grateful to YOU.